100 Questions & Answers About Anxiety

by Laura L. Smith, PhD

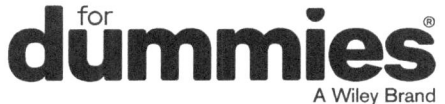

for
dummies®
A Wiley Brand

100 Questions & Answers About Anxiety For Dummies®

Published by: **John Wiley & Sons, Inc.**, 111 River Street, Hoboken, NJ 07030-5774, www.wiley.com

For general information on our other products and services, please contact our Customer Care Department within the U.S. at 877-762-2974, outside the U.S. at 317-572-3993, or fax 317-572-4002. For technical support, please visit https://hub.wiley.com/community/support/dummies.

Wiley publishes in a variety of print and electronic formats and by print-on-demand. Some material included with standard print versions of this book may not be included in e-books or in print-on-demand. If this book refers to media that is not included in the version you purchased, you may download this material at http://booksupport.wiley.com. For more information about Wiley products, visit www.wiley.com.

Library of Congress Control Number is available from the publisher.

ISBN 978-1-394-36878-5 (pbk); ISBN 978-1-394-36881-5 (ebk); ISBN 978-1-394-36880-8 (ebk)

Contents at a Glance

Table of Contents

Introduction

Anxiety is the most common mental health disorder. According to the National Alliance on Mental Illness, about 19 percent of American adults have an anxiety disorder, and about 7 percent of children ages 3 to 17 have anxiety every year. I wrote this book to answer common questions about anxiety — what it is, what causes it, how it differs from everyday worry, and the treatment options available.

About This Book

This book is a reference, which means you don't need to read the chapters in order from beginning to end and you don't have to remember anything — there isn't a test at the end of it.

Within this book, you may note that some web addresses break across two lines of text. If you're reading this book in print and want to visit one of these web pages, simply key in the web address exactly as it's noted in the text, pretending as though the line break doesn't exist. If you're reading this as an e-book, you've got it easy — just click the web address to be taken directly to the web page.

Foolish Assumptions

In writing this book, I made just a couple of assumptions about you, the reader:

» You have anxiety or know someone who has anxiety.

» You have questions, and you want answers.

If those basic assumptions apply to you, you've come to the right place.

Icon Used in This Book

This book uses the following icon in the margins:

TIP

When you see the Tip icon, you'll find information that will make your life a little easier, at least when it comes to anxiety.

Where to Go from Here

If you aren't sure where to begin, head to the Table of Contents and skim through the questions until you find one that catches your eye. Or, if you have a specific topic in mind, search for it in the Index. Want to know absolutely everything? Turn the page and start in with Part 1.

1

Understanding Anxiety

This part explains what anxiety is, its impact on people's lives, and the risk factors for developing it. It also walks you through the physical symptoms of anxiety and helps you recognize anxiety episodes. If you've recently received a diagnosis of anxiety, this part is for you.

Chapter **1**

Introducing Anxiety

There's plenty to worry about — wars, poverty, natural disasters, bird flu, civil unrest, violence, crime, and terrorism threaten the safety and security of people around the world. But most people find that these huge existential threats aren't what keeps them up at night. Instead, it's whether they paid the electric bill, who's going to pick up the kids, or figuring out how to get day-to-day things accomplished. This chapter looks at anxiety — what it is and what it isn't. It describes the types of anxiety disorders and the prevalence of anxiety.

What Is Anxiety?

Anxiety is a feeling in your body that signals fear and distress. You respond to a physical feeling — maybe an increased heart rate, a sinking feeling in your gut, a tightening in your throat, increased sweating, tightness in your chest, or dizziness.

People experience anxiety differently, but the signal those feelings induce are worry, fear, apprehension, or uneasiness. The primary reaction to anxiety is to avoid what you fear. Anxiety is a perfectly normal reaction, until it becomes excessive.

How Is Anxiety Different from Everyday Worry?

In many ways, anxiety and everyday worry are the same. Worry involves physical, behavioral, and emotional responses to something feared — and so does anxiety. People worry about real, probable, possibilities.

When worry becomes severe or persistent, or when it interferes with daily life, it is considered an anxiety disorder.

What Is Generalized Anxiety Disorder?

Generalized anxiety disorder (GAD) is like the common cold of mental health issues. Life causes everyone to worry. But people with GAD worry almost constantly. They worry about their family, even when the worry is unjustified. They worry about money, even when they have enough money in their bank accounts. They worry about the weather, even when it's sunny.

In other words, people with GAD worry about everything, including worry. Why do they worry so much? Because they want to control their environment, their health, and other people's problems, and they want to find solutions. They can't stand the uncertainties of life.

Everyone worries, sometimes too much. But those with GAD can't stop worrying. That worry interferes with their lives and health.

Are There Different Types of Anxiety Disorders?

There are different categories of anxiety. Here are the most common:

» **GAD:** Worry about almost everything all the time.

» **Specific phobia:** A *phobia* (intense fear) of one or more things or situations, such as animals, flying, elevators, heights, vomiting, blood, or just about anything. Avoidance is very strong. Some people have multiple phobias.

» **Social anxiety disorder (also known as social phobia):** Fear of one or more social situations, such as public speaking, interacting with others at a party, meeting new people, or eating and drinking around others. The fear usually relates to worries about being judged by others and is persistent. It also causes avoidance of social situations.

» **Panic disorder:** A quick surge of physical feelings of panic, including shortness of breath, rapid pulse, chest tightness or pain, tremors, nausea, fear of losing control, chills, or feeling feverish. These unexpected attacks start a cycle of worry and attempts to avoid future attacks.

» **Agoraphobia:** Extreme worry about two of the following situations: being outside of the home, standing in a crowded place, being in enclosed spaces (like a theater or shop), being in open spaces (such as a parking lot or mall), or using public transportation.

How Common Is Anxiety?

Anxiety is the most common of all mental disorders. It affects people all over the world. About one in four people have anxiety and about half will suffer from anxiety sometime during their lifetimes. Anxiety is perfectly normal when it's a response to something dangerous or difficult. If you can't pay your bills, you worry. If your teen is out late at night, you become anxious. When a snake is rattling its tail at you, you get scared. Anxiety only becomes a disorder when it is excessive and disrupts everyday life.

Chapter **2**

The Impact of Anxiety

Although everyday stress is the biggest trigger for anxiety, it's only one factor. Other, bigger problems can also cause anxiety (for example, the loss of an important person in your life, a move to a new neighborhood, a potential nuclear war, a flood, or any other natural disaster). Let's face it, the world is one big creator of worry.

No wonder anxiety is by far the most common mental illness. Unfortunately, only about a third of people get help for managing anxiety. Although everyone experiences some anxiety, for those who experience anxiety chronically, the costs are great.

In this chapter, I cover the many effects of anxiety. These include health concerns, difficulty concentrating, memory problems, changes in appetite, and problems with sleeping.

What Are the Long-Term Effects of Untreated Anxiety?

The body's fight-or-flight response is perfectly intended to push through danger. However, if that danger signal is left on for too much of the day and real danger doesn't exist, then the preparation itself leads to chronic illness. Here are some common long-term effects of untreated anxiety:

» High blood pressure

» Heart disease

» Heart palpitations

» Stomach disorders, such as pain, nausea, gas, diarrhea, or ulcers

» Irritable bowel syndrome (IBS)

» Muscle tension, including back pain, neck pain, headaches, and migraines

» Teeth grinding

» Weakened immune system

How Does Anxiety Affect Cognitive Functioning?

The brain takes in information through sight, taste, smell, sound, and touch. The normal brain does a pretty good job at doing that. It usually sees reality. However, the anxious brain is skewed — it may not see things as they are. When a brain is anxious, it takes in information that could very well be good or neutral and interprets it as dangerous. For example, when you're anxious, you may misplace your keys and be absolutely sure that you left them on top of your car and drove off, losing them forever. Then when you find them in your pocket, you feel a great sense of relief.

Anxiety, because of its effect on the brain, impairs *executive functioning* (the ability to plan ahead or solve problems), *processing speed* (the speed at which you take in information), and *cognitive control* (the ability to regulate your emotions and focus).

Can Anxiety Cause Problems with Decision-Making, Attention, Concentration, and Memory?

When your brain is clouded by anxiety, decision-making can be skewed toward a negative bias. For example, say an opportunity to make a good investment becomes available. Even if your financial advisor, who you completely trust, tells you it's safe, your feeling of distress and worry makes you reluctant to take the very low risk to invest. The fear of uncertainty makes an easy decision impossible.

Attention and concentration are also negatively impacted by anxiety. When your brain senses a threat, it automatically focuses all attention on that threat. This may make it impossible to take in other information that may reduce the threat. For example, a veteran with post-traumatic stress disorder (PTSD) may startle when hearing loud noises in the environment (for example, at a fireworks show). The veteran's previous fear experience in war clouds their ability to be able to focus on the present moment.

Memory is also negatively affected by anxiety. When the chemicals of anxiety are flowing through your brain, your ability to hold onto information in your memory is disrupted. You may also forget much of what's happening around you because of your attention to the stressful event. Plus, you may be unable to recall details of the events that are happening.

How Does Anxiety Affect Appetite and Eating?

Anxiety has multiple implications for appetite and eating. People with anxiety may:

- » Overeat to suppress feelings.
- » Lose their appetite completely.
- » Eat only sweets or carbs.
- » Suffer from diarrhea immediately after eating or when they become anxious.
- » Suffer from nausea or vomiting.

TIP

If anxiety causes you to gain or lose weight or eat unhealthy food, your primary care doctor can help you find treatment.

What Symptoms of Anxiety Are Most Disruptive to Daily Life?

All symptoms of anxiety can be disruptive. Who would want to live with a constant feeling of being on edge, worried, fearful, and physically uncomfortable? However, probably the most disturbing symptom of anxiety is the panic attack. During severe attacks, people often go to the emergency room (ER) feeling like they may be having a heart attack.

About 75 percent of those with panic attacks have visited the ER at least once. Remarkably, about a third of all those with severe chest pain in the ER who are not having heart attacks are having panic attacks.

Is Anxiety Always a Bad Thing?

Anxiety, like all emotions, is a signal that something is amiss — but it isn't always a bad thing. If you feel anxious, there may be a good reason. Anxiety tells you to look around for danger, or see if someone is trying to take advantage of you.

But if you're anxious about things that aren't real, or remote possibilities that haven't yet happened, your signal isn't working accurately. That means that you become anxious about something that isn't dangerous or that may or may not happen in the future. Treatment for anxiety resets those faulty signals.

Chapter **3**

Risk Factors for Anxiety

Everyone has times of anxiety. It's as normal as the feeling you get before you jump into a cold swimming pool or take an exam at school. People get anxious about buying and selling houses, having a baby, or getting married. They also get anxious when a forest fire is getting close to their homes, they divorce, they have a baby, or they lose a loved one. These are all normal life events, and anxiety is a perfectly appropriate emotion.

Anxiety disorders are when the level of anxiety is more than expected, it interferes with daily living, and increases the risk of depression. This chapter details factors that increase the chances of normal anxiety developing into a problem.

How Does Anxiety Typically Develop over Time?

Anxiety disorders often start in childhood or adolescence. But adults can also develop anxiety. Whatever the time of life or the cause. There is a cycle of anxiety.

That cycle is something like an itch. If you have an itch from a mosquito bite, you scratch it and feel an instantaneous sense of relief. But soon after you scratch that itch, it almost always returns.

With anxiety, you feel anxious, you try to find ways to quell those bad feelings. Maybe you go home and stay away from a party, maybe you stay away from a challenging job opportunity, maybe you try worrying about what might happen in the future. None of those temporary fixes work. You're left with more anxiety. That's why most anxiety disorders start out minor and get worse over time.

Can Anyone Develop Anxiety?

Anyone can develop anxiety. Even dogs and cats can be anxious. If you're walking in a dark alley and you hear a scream, who wouldn't be anxious? If you know that a hurricane is heading your way, it's a good idea to worry enough to make necessary preparations.

However, most people don't develop an anxiety disorder after having a fearful experience. An anxiety disorder develops over time; often other factors such as family history and trauma interact.

Remember: Anxiety is a natural reaction to stress or fear. It only becomes a disorder when there's nothing to really be anxious about and the anxiety causes you to not be able to carry out your normal everyday tasks.

Is Anxiety Hereditary?

Anxiety tends to run in families, but heredity doesn't appear to be a major cause. Studies of twins suggest that genetics may play a part in developing anxiety. For example, identical twins are more likely to both have anxiety than fraternal twins or siblings. It's estimated that somewhere between 30 percent and 60 percent of anxiety is related to heredity. When heredity mixes with other factors, anxiety may be more likely to emerge.

How Can Your Upbringing Cause Anxiety?

If you have a parent with an anxiety disorder, you're about seven times more likely to develop an anxiety disorder. Is that genetic or something else?

Consider this. Say your mother worries about germs. She's constantly washing your hands and face, telling you that you might get sick from touching something. You may learn that same behavior and feel stressed about getting dirty.

Or maybe your father is incredibly shy and stays home most of the time. Because he stays home, you stay home and don't learn to be social with other people. Is that genetic or learned? It could be both.

What Is the Relationship between Trauma and Anxiety?

Millions of people experience trauma. Trauma comes in many forms, from natural disasters to violent crime. Childhood trauma involves abuse, severe neglect, or loss. All these factors increase the likelihood of developing anxiety. Different people respond differently to trauma. Some experience anxiety; others quickly recover. Personal characteristics and temperament may lead to decreased or increased sensitivity to traumatic events.

TIP

There has been a change in the use of the word *trauma* over time. Many everyday stressors — for example, a toxic boss or a disloyal friend — are identified as "traumatic." These events, though difficult to deal with, are not considered traumatic enough on their own to cause an anxiety disorder.

Are Certain Temperaments More Prone to Anxiety than Others?

If you've spent time with babies or little kids, you may have noticed that some are pretty laid back — they cry when they're hungry or tired, but otherwise they're content — whereas others are clingy and easily disturbed. Many studies suggest that kids are born with certain temperaments.

These traits either protect or predict later trouble with anxiety. Here are some of the characteristics that may spell trouble:

>> Being shy and withdrawing in new situations

>> Displaying emotions such as sadness, fear, or anger quickly and because of small frustrations

>> Being introverted or very slow to warm up

>> Resisting trying new activities

>> Being cautious and fearful of getting hurt

All these tendencies can change over time. With good role models and understanding adults, these early temperamental traits can turn into strengths.

Chapter **4**

Physical Manifestations of Anxiety

How do you know that you're feeling anxious? Maybe you find yourself repeatedly going over a worry. You're fearful of something that may happen in the future, or you avoid going out of your house. Along with thinking and behaving, anxiety almost always involves a physical component. These physical symptoms are often the first clues that anxiety is lurking around the corner.

Can Anxiety Affect Physical Health?

Anxiety can absolutely affect physical health. The initial physical reaction to anxiety starts almost immediately. Anxiety causes the body to go into a fight-or-flight response — the body is ready to either fight off the danger or run away from it. Therefore, the brain sends a message to the nervous system to go on high alert.

Immediately, the heart starts beating faster and harder. The blood flow increases to the large muscle groups for better running, kicking, or hitting. Lungs fill with more oxygen, muscles tense, and sweating increases, keeping the body cool and slippery so that the predator can't hold on. Blood flow to the hands and feet decrease and digestion stops. Chronic anxiety leads to a variety of physical problems.

What Are the Most Common Physical Symptoms of Anxiety?

When they're anxious, many people start to take rapid, short breaths, which can induce a feeling of dizziness. Then, the brain sends out signals to increase the production of activating chemicals, making you feel out of breath or increasing your heart rate. The initial burst of anxiety spirals and grows.

In addition, many people with anxiety develop an upset stomach with nausea and diarrhea. You may also experience a choking sensation.

Muscles often tense up, which can lead to headaches, back pain, or neck pain. You may feel sweaty or overwhelmingly tired. Constant worry can also lead to insomnia.

What Does Anxiety Do to the Body over Time?

Over time, untreated anxiety often leads to *depression,* a serious disease that involves loss of pleasure in life, hopelessness, helplessness, and sometimes suicidal thoughts or behaviors.

Another problem with untreated anxiety is that many people find other ways to manage their discomfort, including drinking to excess, engaging in disturbed eating (for example, eating a gallon of ice cream or barely eating at all), smoking too much marijuana, abusing prescription medications, or taking illegal drugs. Sleep problems increase the chances of misusing over-the-counter medications or becoming dependent on a prescription sleep medication.

Can Your Body Be Anxious without You Feeling Anxious?

Your body can feel agitated or restless without you realizing why. Other physical symptoms — such as stomach upset, muscle tightness, and increased heart rate — may also be present.

This condition is generally known as *subconscious anxiety.* Your brain may be processing messages that you're unaware of consciously. For example, perhaps you encounter someone who resembles the person who traumatized you in early in childhood, causing your body to react even if you don't recall the event. Or maybe your worry about paying bills spills into the present moment when you're busy with something else. That worry may be constant despite what you're doing.

Can Anxiety Cause Stomach Problems?

Doctors once believed that a condition called irritable bowel syndrome (IBS) was caused by stress, worry, and anxiety. That belief is now questioned, but the answers aren't clear. Did anxiety cause IBS, or did IBS cause anxiety?

Either way, people with IBS suffer from cramps and pain in the digestive system. They either have bouts of diarrhea or constipation, and often both. Treatment relieves symptoms. Psychotherapy that teaches stress relief strategies also helps.

Can Anxiety Cause Chronic Pain?

The relationship between chronic pain and anxiety is multifaceted. Anxiety can directly cause chronic pain primarily because of muscle tightness, which can lead to pain in the neck or back or frequent headaches. Anxiety also leads to increased pain perception. In other words, if you have pain, anxiety makes it *more* painful. Chronic pain can also lead to more anxiety and stress. In addition, it can interfere with sleep, making both the pain and the anxiety worse.

Can Anxiety Cause Dizziness or Excessive Sweating?

Anxiety causes dizziness because of the increased heart rate and the act of taking shallow, quick breaths. That leads to feeling lightheaded. Like chronic pain, the relationship between anxiety and dizziness is bidirectional — when someone feels dizzy, they're likely to feel even more anxious. So, there is a reciprocal relationship between the two.

The two hormones released when you're anxious are cortisol and adrenaline. These hormones increase the sweat response. Again, sweating often increases the feeling of anxiety. Sweaty palms often occur without a conscious feeling of anxiety.

Use the information your body is giving you to take some deep breaths and consider what's making you anxious.

TIP

Can Anxiety Raise My Blood Pressure?

When you're anxious, because of the release of hormones, your blood pressure will likely rise. It should return to normal when the anxiety decreases. Some people have what's called *white-coat syndrome* (high blood pressure that occurs in the doctor's office). If that happens to you, your provider will likely ask you to monitor your blood pressure at home or in other settings.

Chronic anxiety may eventually result in chronic high blood pressure. So, it's important to get help if you have chronic anxiety.

How Can I Tell the Difference between Anxiety and Another Physical Reaction?

It's not always easy to tell the difference. Multiple physical problems mimic feelings that cause someone to think they may be anxious. Here are a few examples of conditions and possible symptoms:

» **Low blood sugar:** Clammy feeling, sweating, confusion, rapid heartbeat

» **Hyperthyroidism:** Nervousness, restlessness, fatigue, tremor, diarrhea

» **Other hormonal imbalances:** Tension, irritability, headaches, mood swings, fatigue, panic

» **Heart disease:** Shortness of breath, rapid breathing, chest tightness or pain, skipped heartbeats, feeling like you're not getting enough air

» **Chronic lung conditions such as chronic obstructive pulmonary disease (COPD) or asthma:** Feeling like you're not able to get enough air, shortness of breath, tightness in the chest, panic

Other conditions also have symptoms of anxiety. If you develop anxiety and don't know why, it's a good idea to check with your primary care provider to rule out possible causes.

Chapter **5**

Recognizing Anxiety Episodes

Anxiety prepares people to stomp on the breaks when the car in front of them unexpectedly stops, or pull a child out of danger when they're carelessly wandering into the bike lane on a hike. It helps keep people safe, prepared, and ready to act.

However, anxiety is out of control when it occurs for too long or happens when there is no external danger. In this chapter, I describe various forms and symptoms of disordered anxiety.

What Are the Signs of an Anxiety Attack?

An anxiety attack involves overwhelming anxiety or worry. There is usually a cause, such as an impending public speech, a meeting with your boss, an argument with your ex, or selling your house.

This threat causes anxiety to gradually build over time. Sometimes you may feel intense symptoms; other times, your anxiety decreases when you're distracted. Physical symptoms may include sweating, a racing heart, and difficulty concentrating.

What Is a Panic Attack?

A panic attack appears out of the blue. It tends to be sudden and is characterized by mainly physical, intense feelings. Your heart may pound and race, your muscles may tighten, you may sweat occurs, and you may be overwhelmed by a great feeling of doom. People having panic attacks feel like they're suffocating and have shortness of breath. Panic attacks often feel like heart attacks, so people end up in the emergency room. Panic attacks generally last only a few minutes.

Panic attacks lead to a great fear of having another panic attack. That leads to more anxiety. There are many good treatments for panic and anxiety (see Parts 3 and 4 for more information).

How Does Chronic Anxiety Differ from Acute Anxiety?

Chronic anxiety stays with you over a long period of time. People with chronic anxiety tend to worry about almost everything. They have a constant state of tension and feel restless or on edge. Chronic anxiety also leads to tension headaches, an upset stomach, and other physical symptoms. People with chronic anxiety worry about things that are extremely unlikely to happen or impossible to prepare for, such as "What if a meteor hits the earth tomorrow?"

Acute anxiety involves sudden bursts of feelings that generally abate when the stressor is removed. A panic attack is an example of acute anxiety. It comes on suddenly and usually goes away quickly.

What Symptoms Indicate That Normal Anxiety Is Becoming a Disorder?

Anxiety is a normal response to novel situations. For example, someone may be very nervous at a job interview. Usually, as time passes, the initial anxiety decreases, and the person becomes more comfortable.

Normal anxiety always passes with time. Disordered anxiety continues even after the trigger has passed. For example, after a minor car accident, everyone involved is usually anxious. But if a person stops driving because of a fender bender, that becomes disordered anxiety.

Can Anxiety Symptoms Fluctuate over Time?

Anxiety symptoms can fluctuate. Stress from outside can increase anxiety quickly. If you have an anxiety disorder and you lose your job, end a relationship, experience financial stress, or have an argument, your anxiety spikes.

And anxiety can decrease when the outside world provides a pleasurable distraction or you feel less stress in your life.

Is Avoiding Situations over Fear a Symptom of Anxiety?

Avoidance is a major feature of anxiety. People with social anxiety avoid public speaking, parties, or large crowds. People with panic disorder avoid things they believe may make them panic. And people with phobias avoid whatever they're afraid of (for example, leaving the house, flying, elevators, spiders, snakes, and so on).

Anxious people avoid taking risks that may benefit them, such as a job promotion, a special relationship, or a creative task. They don't want to take the chance that they may be judged as a failure or inadequate.

Are There Lesser-Known Symptoms That May Indicate an Anxiety Disorder?

When you're anxious, hormones surge through your body and may cause some uncommon symptoms. For example, you may yawn excessively. That's because your breathing may become shallow, so the body reacts by yawning to increase the levels of oxygen.

Another symptom thought to be caused by anxiety is temperature changes, usually in the face, feet, or hands. The face or extremities can experience either excessive heat or coldness.

Feelings of numbness, tingling, or trembling also sometimes occur with anxiety.

Finally, *dissociation* (the feeling that you're disconnected from reality) can occur with severe anxiety, usually associated with trauma. It may involve loss of memory of the current stress or trauma, or feeling as if it were a dream and avoiding painful feelings. Dissociation is a coping mechanism when someone is overwhelmed by anxiety.

2

Causes and Triggers of Anxiety

This part outlines how anxiety differs among various groups of people, the physical and biological triggers of anxiety, and how environmental factors and stress affect anxiety. It also dives into conditions that can occur alongside anxiety.

Chapter **6**

Anxiety across Ages and Cultures

Anxiety is unique for every person, yet there are similarities among groups. This chapter looks at ages and stages of anxiety, cultural differences, sex differences, and their relationship to anxiety.

How Does Anxiety Differ across the Lifespan?

During childhood, anxiety may look quite different than in adulthood. Anxious children may have temper tantrums when they want to avoid something that they fear. They may throw up or act hyperactive or irritable. *Phobias* (fears of specific things) often begin in childhood.

Throughout adulthood, all anxiety disorders remain, with symptoms increasing and decreasing over time.

In late adulthood, seniors sometimes develop generalized anxiety. They become worried about their health and independence. Anxiety also shows up with dementia and is part of the disease process.

Are There Any Unique Symptoms of Anxiety in Children?

Two types of anxiety are generally found exclusively in children: separation anxiety and selective mutism.

Separation anxiety involves intense worry about separation from parents or caregivers. This type of anxiety is commonly found in young children, but when it continues to school age, it can be a particularly difficult problem.

The other anxiety disorder primarily occurring with children is much rarer than separation anxiety. *Selective mutism* is the refusal to speak in any situation that arouses anxiety. Kids with selective mutism are silent with most people outside of their families. This form of anxiety causes massive social and educational consequences.

Does Anxiety Differ in Women and Men?

Women are almost *twice* as likely to experience an anxiety disorder, with one exception: Social anxiety is equally distributed among men and women. Age of onset of anxiety and how long the disorder remains are similar.

Women more often use avoidance to deal with anxiety. Men are more likely to abuse substances in response to anxiety.

How Do Cultural Factors Influence Anxiety?

Culture affects the way anxiety is expressed. In some cultures, anxiety produces primarily physical symptoms; in others, rumination or constant worry goes along with anxiety.

Anxiety can also be a product of social stigma against certain groups, such as immigrants and people of color. For example, young Black men are warned about the importance of being extremely passive and polite when they're interacting with police — a result of years of discrimination and violence perpetuated by racism.

How Does a Person's Upbringing Influence Anxiety Levels Later in Life?

Parents or other caregivers influence children through role modeling. Children look to important adults in their lives and learn from what they do, how they react, and how they think about things.

For example, if your parents were constantly worried about paying the bills, you may have grown up with a similar stance about finances. You may constantly fret about bill paying or saving enough money for retirement.

Some adults become frantically anxious about travel. When packing for a trip, they're obsessed with making sure they have everything they'll need. If you had that kind of role model as a child, you may find yourself getting anxious about travel or forgetting something, too.

TIP

Role models act as teachers, but you can unlearn your role models' bad anxiety habits.

Chapter **7**

Biological and Internal Triggers

This chapter delves deeper into the physical and biological factors related to anxiety. Triggers can be either external or internal. For example, an external trigger that produces anxiety could be a traffic ticket and the worry of added expense on car insurance. An internal trigger leading to increased anxiety could be a feeling of being on edge caused by too much coffee.

Why Is Anxiety Often Thought of as a Physical and Emotional Disorder?

With depression, you can feel fatigue or restlessness and have problems with eating or sleeping, but depression is primarily a disease of negative thinking and sad, hopeless feelings.

Anxiety, on the other hand, *always* involves a physical component. Whether it's shakiness, tight muscles, a lump in the stomach, dizziness, a racing heart, or something else, anxiety is primarily a change in body functioning along with emotional responses of worry, fear, or disgust.

How Do Hormones and Brain Chemistry Impact Anxiety?

Hormones such as insulin, thyroxine, estrogen, cortisol, and testosterone are released by the endocrine glands (which include the thyroid, pituitary, and adrenal glands). Hormones communicate with the body and can influence mood, including anxiety. Problems with the thyroid gland, for example, can directly cause feeling of anxiety; too much cortisol also increases anxiety.

Brain chemicals, such as serotonin, acetylcholine, dopamine, and gamma-aminobutyric acid (GABA), travel across nerve cells and communicate information. All these chemicals work together.

A popular concept is that a chemical imbalance of brain chemistry is responsible for mental health disorders. The problem is, no one really knows how that works. Evidence comes from the successful management of anxiety through the use of medications that change the availability of particular brain chemicals.

Can Anxiety Be Triggered by Certain Foods or Drinks?

Probably the most common drinks that increase anxiety are energy drinks. Loaded with caffeine and other stimulants such as guarana, ginseng, taurine, and sugar, energy drinks can definitely cause restlessness and jitteriness. In some cases, they can be dangerous if overconsumed.

Sugar can also cause anxiety when overconsumed. Have you ever watched the way kids act after a sugar-laden birthday party? Adults can have the same reaction.

Some people suffer from specific food sensitivities. If you seem to feel more anxious after eating or drinking a particular food, try tracking it for a few weeks. It may be best to eliminate that food from your diet.

How Does Sleep Affect Anxiety?

Lack of sleep seems to make everything worse. If you don't get enough sleep or if the quality of your sleep is poor, the problems of your world can quickly seem overwhelmingly unsolvable. Getting a good night's sleep for a few nights in a row makes your thoughts settle down, and realistic, logical thinking becomes possible.

Anxiety makes your sleep worse. Tossing and turning with anxious thoughts is a common complaint of those who suffer from anxiety. It's a vicious cycle — and another reminder why sleep is so important.

How Does Hydration Affect Anxiety Levels?

Dehydration increases feelings of anxiety. For example, when you're dehydrated, you may feel weak and dizzy, which causes concern and worry. Dehydration also affects hormones and brain chemistry, which can increase anxious feelings. Finally, dehydration may sometimes be related to a feeling of panic, resulting in a full panic attack.

Can Physical Health Conditions Trigger Anxiety?

Having a health condition, especially if it's chronic, can increase anxiety. Some conditions, however, are especially likely to cause anxiety. Here are some examples:

» **Hypoglycemia:** Low blood sugar can cause confusion, trembling, irritability, rapid heartbeat, weakness, cold, and clammy feelings.

» **Hyperthyroidism:** Too much thyroid hormone can result in restlessness, sweating, diarrhea, tremors, racing heartbeat, and nervousness.

» **Heart disease:** Heart disease can lead to shortness of breath, chest pain or tightness, and skipped or irregular heartbeats.

» **Chronic lung conditions:** Asthma, chronic obstructive pulmonary disease (COPD), or other lung diseases cause a feeling of not getting enough air, shortness of breath, tightness in the chest, and panic.

Chapter **8**

Environmental Factors, Stress, and Anxiety

Today the world seems more stressful than the "good old days." You're bombarded with information and choices — from what to watch on the myriad streaming platforms to breaking news. And all that information is on your phone 24/7. Stress turns to anxiety when it lingers and starts to interfere with getting things done.

Can Anxiety Be Triggered by Environmental Factors?

Anxiety and stress swell when temperatures go up. So do tempers. Constant noise — such as busy freeways, barking dogs, music blasting, or frequent loud arguments among housemates or neighbors — escalates anxiety. Sudden, piercing, but fairly frequent noise — such as explosions or gunshots in an actual war or in a neighborhood with gunshots and fights — can lead to anxiety, too.

Other factors such as air pollution, lack of resources, poor water supply, harsh lighting, and poverty intensify stress and anxiety.

Earthquakes, hurricanes, floods, forest fires, tornadoes, landslides, tsunamis, and volcanic eruptions all can lead to anxiety. However, it's not considered a disorder if recovery takes place after the issues are cleaned up and resolved.

Interestingly, getting out in nature is a remedy for anxiety and stress. Research indicates that sitting outside in a pleasant park or outside recreation is a good antidote to stress.

Are Certain Lifestyles or Habits More Likely to Lead to Anxiety?

Lifestyle and habits can amplify anxiety. Here are a few common ones:

» **Being overscheduled:** People who can't say no end up with too many responsibilities and not enough time to complete them.

» **Feeling bored:** Boredom can amplify anxiety. When people don't have a purpose, they often spend time worrying.

» **Poor organization:** When a person's life, home, and work environment are a mess, it's hard to focus on the important tasks.

» **Always running late:** Some people, no matter how much time they have to get ready, can't get out the door on time. They're rushing to work, to the airport, or to another function. Being late escalates stress and anxiety.

» **Being the partner of someone who is always late:** It's hard to adjust and accept when your partner is late, which makes you share the stress.

» **Procrastinating:** People who procrastinate push the limits of being able to get finished on time. This adds stress and anxiety to every put-off task.

How Does Social Media Impact Anxiety?

Teens and young adults have more depression and anxiety than ever before. Many researchers believe there's a direct connection between rising rates of mental illness and time spent on social media.

The more time spent on social media, the more likely a young person is to become socially withdrawn, anxious, and depressed. Teenagers spend an average of about five hours a day on social media. Millennials spend a bit less (three hours).

Why does the correlation between time on social media and anxiety appear to be so strong?

» **Along with other life necessities, time on social media leaves little time to socialize with real-life friends.** Indeed, teenagers are spending far less time going out and much more time staying home than previous generations did.

» **Spending time on social media can make teenagers (and adults, too!) feel like everybody else is having more fun.** Most people only post photos or videos them-selves doing exciting or positive activities. You see people having parties, families on vacation, as well as touched-up glamour shots. When you believe that you don't measure up on social media, you may feel bad about yourself and your life.

» **According to the United Nations, about a third of all young people have experienced some form of cyberbullying.** *Cyberbullying* is often willfully repeated, malicious, threatening, or humiliating information sent across social media plat-forms. This type of bullying can increase anxiety. Unfortunately, a few adolescents have actually committed suicide as the result of this form of abuse.

Does Social Pressure Lead to Anxiety?

Social pressure (the belief that you should act, look, achieve, or conform to an expectation) frequently leads to anxiety. If someone doesn't meet those expectations, they may believe that they're judged as not good enough.

There is tremendous social pressure to achieve a certain level of financial success. Those who are unable to achieve that feel victimized and criticized by others.

Youth and beauty are very powerful examples of social pressure. When time inevitably moves on, a multi-billion-dollar industry steps in to help. Not feeling young or beautiful enough makes people feel that they aren't good enough overall, which can lead to feelings of inadequacy and anxiousness.

There are strong pushes to follow the norms of society. When someone doesn't conform, they may fear being judged. This leads to feeling out of place and anxious.

Can Major Life Changes Trigger Anxiety?

Major changes can trigger anxiety. However, the amount of stress caused by change varies from person to person. For example, a young person going out on a date may become extremely anxious over the eruption of a blemish. A 55-year-old overweight man may get anxious when he finds himself out of breath after climbing a flight of stairs.

Here are some common stressors that may cause you anxiety:

» Death of a partner or other loved one
» Divorce or separation
» Major illness or injury
» Going to jail or prison
» Loss of a job
» Retirement
» Birth of a child
» Starting a new job
» Financial stress
» Buying or selling a house

How Does Financial Stress Impact Anxiety?

Everyone needs a certain amount of income for survival. But people who can survive also worry about money — money for rent, for food, for presents for the kids. They worry about credit card debt or not saving enough for retirement or a rainy-day fund.

General worry about finances is perfectly normal. However, if the worry paralyzes you, makes you constantly anxious, or interferes with your happiness and ability to take on daily obligations, it has become a source of anxiety.

TIP

To approach this overwhelming sense of anxiety, start by getting someone to help you go over your budget. Do you have good reasons to be alarmed? If so, credit agencies can help. If your worries are mainly unrealistic, ask your primary-care provider for a referral to a mental health professional.

How Does Work-Related Stress Contribute to Anxiety?

Stress is a temporary reaction to something that is challenging, annoying, unfair, or abusive. Work stress occurs when the work environment, whether the job expectations or interpersonal relations, become difficult to manage.

Work stress leads to anxiety when it's chronic and solutions are not apparent. When the anxiety bleeds into time sleeping, loss of appetite, and irritability at home as well as work, seek out treatment.

How Do Personal Relationships Affect Anxiety Levels?

People close to you have a significant impact on anxiety. Depending on how close you are, the impact can be very significant. For example, if you live with someone who is unsupportive, argumentative, and dismissive, anxiety levels will likely rise.

On the other hand, if your partner is supportive and understanding, that may help you feel more grounded and less anxious.

One kind of support is toxic: Partners who are overly protective, give constant reassurance, and have the need to baby their anxious partner usually make their partner worse. That's because the anxious partner leans too much on their protective partner and becomes weaker and less confident.

How Does Perfectionism Contribute to Anxiety?

If you must be perfect, that's pretty stressful. Perfectionists believe that either something is perfect and right or it's worthless, and the consequences will be devastating.

They ruminate over small, sometimes unimportant details. When they make a mistake, they blame themselves and feel horrible. Their parents probably told them if something's worth doing, it's worth doing perfectly.

Chapter **9**

Comorbidities and Related Conditions

Comorbidities are quite common in all mental disorders. Generally, comorbidities make both conditions worse and harder to treat. Treatment becomes more challenging, and outcomes are often quite poor. Some experts believe that there is a genetic component that is related to both anxiety and depression that make some people more susceptible to both.

This chapter explores the relationship between anxiety and a host of other problems.

Is Irritability a Sign of Anxiety?

When you think about any mental disorder, including anxiety, it helps to visualize that it takes up considerable room in your brain to be anxious. Therefore, you just can't take on much more. Small frustrations cause eruptions of irritability. You may snap at someone because anxiety is flooding out your ability to control your negative emotions.

In other words, you're just more vulnerable and emotionally sensitive when anxious.

Do Anxiety Disorders Coexist with Other Disorders?

Anxiety often coexists with other anxiety disorders. For example, someone with generalized anxiety (constant worry) may also suffer from social anxiety. Someone with panic disorder may easily develop *agoraphobia* (fear of leaving the house). Like all comorbid mental health problems, having more than one at a time makes treatment more difficult.

Anxiety can also coexist with depression, chronic pain, substance abuse disorders, post-traumatic stress disorder (PTSD), and obsessive-compulsive disorder (OCD). Again, when more than one disorder exists, treatment is more complicated and self-harm becomes a real concern.

What Is the Relationship between Anxiety and OCD?

Both anxiety and OCD involve anxiety. In fact, OCD used to be categorized as a form of an anxiety disorder. Now, OCD is thought to be different enough that it has its own category.

OCD involves intrusive thoughts, urges, or images (the obsessions) that are frequent and seem to be uncontrollable. Those obsessions lead to discomfort and anxiety and the need to perform a compulsive behavior. Examples of compulsions include handwashing, repeatedly checking that a door is locked or the stove is off, superstitious chanting, cleaning, repeating phrases, arranging things in a specific order or many other actions that make the obsessions go away. However, with OCD the obsessions return, and the pattern repeats itself.

Anxiety does not include obsessions and compulsions. However, you can have both OCD and anxiety.

Can Anxiety Cause Symptoms That Mimic Other Psychological Conditions?

Imagine someone who always says no to invitations and rarely leaves home except for work. Finally, someone convinces them to attend a work function. The person sits quietly, head down; doesn't try to mingle; and leaves early. Maybe they have depression, social phobia, agoraphobia, or chronic pain — you really don't know. So, yes, anxiety can look like other mental disorders, especially depression, PTSD, and OCD.

In addition, anxiety can look like a physical illness. For example, constant digestive symptoms can be caused by anxiety or another disease. Rapid heart rate and shortness of breath could be symptoms of heart disease or anxiety.

TIP

The fact that anxiety can look like other disorders is another reason to get an annual physical and a mental health evaluation.

Are There Warning Symptoms That Anxiety Is Leading to Depression?

When anxiety isn't treated, depression can set in. Symptoms start with irritability, problems sleeping, and changes in eating. Sadness, helplessness, and hopelessness may be present.

A person can feel unable to fix themselves and experience feelings of worthlessness. They retreat even further into their aloneness and lose the sense of pleasure in daily life.

The stress of prolonged anxiety causes loss of pleasure and even loss of self-esteem. An anxious person whose life is limited by anxiety can question why they should bother doing anything. Suicidal thoughts and even attempts are possible.

Can Anxiety Be Caused by Substance Abuse?

When people withdraw from drugs or alcohol, they're very likely to experience severe anxiety. Symptoms include extreme restlessness, feelings of desperation, tremors, sweating, loss of sleep, raised heart rate, agitation, and tension.

These feelings should subside over time if the withdrawal is successful. However, sometimes anxious people turn to drugs or alcohol as a relief from anxiety, and the anxiety returns after the withdrawal without further treatment.

Can Anxiety Be a Side-Effect of Medication?

Medicines prescribed to treat common conditions such as asthma, inflammation, depression, or colds often have side effects that can resemble anxiety. Here are a few examples of these medications:

» Steroids to treat inflammation, arthritis, and pain

» Bronchodilators to treat asthma

» Stimulant medications to treat attention-deficit/hyperactivity disorder (ADHD)

» Thyroid replacement medications to treat hypothyroidism

» Novocain to blocks pain in dentistry

TIP

If you have symptoms of anxiety following a newly prescribed medication, talk to your doctor and pharmacist about possible side effects.

3

Managing Your Anxiety

IN THIS PART . . .

This part offers techniques for managing your anxiety on your own. It provides techniques you can use to immediately reduce your anxiety level and explains how mindfulness and other self-help techniques work. It also offers tips on modifying your lifestyle and environment to manage anxiety and how to get support from family, friends, and others.

Chapter **10**
Immediate Relief Strategies

Chronic anxiety requires treatment, either psychotherapy or medication. However, there are times when short-term solutions can help calm anxiety. This chapter reviews some easy-to-use techniques.

How Can Deep Breathing Help with Anxiety?

Deep breathing is one of my go-to strategies. It works for quelling anxiety, anger management, and keeping yourself from saying something you'll regret later on. You can practice breath work discreetly, so others won't even notice you're doing it. For example, say you're stressed in a social situation. You can take slow deep breaths. You don't need to make noise while doing it, so it can be done anywhere.

Does Meditation Help with Anxiety?

Numerous studies have proven that meditation can decrease the severity of anxiety and improve the ability to cope with stress. In addition, meditation improves sleep, which also decreases anxiety symptoms. Another benefit of meditation is that it improves *working memory* (a type of short-term memory) and may even delay dementia!

There are thousands of meditation practices, so you can find something that works for you. The basic premise is to concentrate on a certain activity — it could be breathing, walking, or even eating.

TIP

The most important thing to remember is that meditation should be an almost everyday practice. Find a ten-minute period in your day, and stick to it!

Are There Certain Phrases or Mantras That Can Calm Anxiety?

Mantras consist of words, phrases, or sounds that are repeated throughout your meditation process. They can calm an anxious mind.

In addition to meditation, you can use affirmations to help you stay calm and focused. For example, repeat to yourself:

» I am capable.
» Breathe and stay calm.
» This feeling will pass.
» Doing this makes me better.
» It gets easier over time.
» This is no big deal — I can handle it.

Are There Any Relaxation Techniques That Can Help Manage Anxiety on the Go?

Progressive muscle relaxation (PMR) is a technique in which you tense and then relax muscle groups throughout your body. You can moderate this whole-muscle approach to any situation. For example, raise and tighten your shoulders, hold for ten seconds, and then let go. Clench your fists, roll your toes, pull in your stomach muscles. These activities can be done discreetly and easily.

Another strategy is to take a short walk outside. Even if the weather is bad, going outside causes your body to readjust, and movement always helps decrease anxiety.

Drink water, brush your teeth, stretch, change up what you're doing. All these quick techniques can help you relax and improve your mood.

What Should I Do If My Anxiety Is Getting Worse?

If you've tried self-help techniques and your anxiety is getting worse, it's time for professional intervention. First, make an appointment with your primary-care provider. Talk to them about your anxiety and make sure it isn't caused by a new medication or a physical condition. After those possibilities are ruled out, ask for a referral to a mental-health professional who specializes in anxiety (see Chapters 14 and 15 for more information).

Chapter **11**
Mindfulness and Self-Help Approaches

Self-help in the form of books, online guides, videos, apps, or support groups can be very useful tools for helping people cope with anxiety. This chapter takes a look at some of those approaches.

At the same time, there are many tools you can pursue yourself to manage your symptoms and decrease your suffering. This chapter describes some of those strategies.

TIP

Some people become even more anxious when trying self-help approaches. They may worry that they aren't trying hard enough or have thoughts about being a failure. If you feel stressed about self-help, don't fret — there's lots of professional help out there. Don't make yourself more anxious about your anxiety.

How Does Mindfulness Help Manage Anxiety?

My dog, Charlie, a goofy goldendoodle, is an expert in mindfulness. Every day she's thrilled with her food, which happens to be the same kibble. Most of the time, her tail is wagging. She loves people, other dogs, treats, and rides in the car.

Charlie hates going to the vet. But until I park the car and get her out, she's happy all the way there. When we get close to the door. She plops her 80-pound self on the ground and doesn't move. However, when one of the techs comes out to help me get her into the office, she responds to the new person with joy. That's because despite her fear of the vet, she can't help but love people. She focuses on what is in front of her in the moment.

When, like most dogs, you stay focused on the present moment, you won't be stressed about the past or the future. Mindfulness means staying focused on what's happening right now.

No worries about the future or guilt about past actions.

Be more in touch with what is happening right now, and you'll learn to be less anxious.

Can Journaling or Expressive Writing Alleviate Anxiety Symptoms?

One relatively easy way to decrease anxiety is keeping a gratitude journal. By thinking about the good things in your life, positive emotions counteract negative emotions. You only have to write a few sentences to have this relatively easy task positively impact your mood.

Sometimes anxiety encourages you to believe that nothing much positive is going on. Take a moment and check out your life. Do you have enough to eat? Can you read? Can you hear birds or smell flowers? Are people ever nice to you? Can you walk, or talk, or think? How about enjoying a good show?

I'll bet you can find something to be grateful for. Give it a try for a couple of weeks and see how you feel.

Do Any Mobile Apps Help Manage Anxiety?

New apps are always coming and going. However, there are a few that have lasted for a while. Before you purchase or subscribe to an app. Check other sources of information about whether the app uses evidence-based practices. You can find reliable reviews on sites such as CNET (www.cnet.com), Healthline (www.healthline.com), Mayo Clinic (www.mayoclinic.org), or WebMD (www.webmd.com).

TIP

Here are some apps I can recommend:

» Calm (www.calm.com)

» Happify (www.happify.com)

» Headspace (www.headspace.com)

» Mindshift CBT (search your device's app store)

» Rootd (www.rootd.io)

» Talkspace (www.talkspace.com)

» Worry Watch (https://worrywatch.com)

Some of these apps connect you with a therapist and some provide lessons or tasks related to anxiety relief. Be sure to access the free trial and check them out before you commit your time and money.

How Does Self-Confidence Help with Anxiety?

Worry and self-confidence act like a seesaw, the more self-confidence you feel, the less worry you have. And the more anxiety you have, the less self-confidence you have.

When you're anxious, you may be worried about a presentation you're making, a job interview, an exam, or showing up at a party. Lots of anxiety involves worrying about performance or being judged. People with high self-esteem tend not to have those worries.

Some people with anxiety spend much of their time worrying about future events such as:

» Will there be another pandemic?
» When will the next disaster hit?
» What happens if I lose my job?
» Will my children grow up happy?

People with high self-esteem tend to believe that whatever happens, they'll do the best they can to manage any future problems.

How Can I Manage Anxiety without Medication?

It's entirely possible to manage anxiety without medication. Almost 60 percent of people with chronic anxiety do not take medication. In fact, the American Medical Association recommends cognitive behavioral therapy as the first choice for treatment (see Chapter 14 for more about therapy).

Part 3 of this book reviews multiple ways to deal with anxiety. If the strategies in this part don't work, check with your primary-care provider about other options.

DID YOU KNOW?

Multitasking, one factor that leads to anxiety, leads to impaired driving. It makes you slower to respond to the traffic ahead, decreases your ability to pay attention, and increases your chance of causing an accident.

Chapter **12**
Lifestyle Adjustments

You may have heard the myth that doing two things at once *increases* productivity or at least decreases boredom. And even if you haven't, the world around us encourages multitasking. Odds are, you check your phone while watching TV or secretly play games while listening to a lecture. One part of your attention is on one thing, but you're also paying attention to something else — and that can increase anxiety.

This chapter describes the many ways that changing lifestyle and habits can help decrease anxiety.

What Are Some Lifestyle Changes That Can Help Reduce Anxiety?

The biggest source of anxiety in today's world is overscheduling. Try to set realistic expectations and reduce anxiety by:

» Not saying yes when you don't have time or interest
» Asking for help when you need it
» Prioritizing your family and yourself
» Knowing your own limitations and sticking to them
» Slowing down and enjoying each moment
» Making time for rejuvenation and joy

How Can I Create a Daily Routine That Helps Mitigate Anxiety?

I have a schedule that includes having coffee, walking the dog, catching up on email and texts, keeping up with the news, working, exercising, meditating, eating healthy, and getting enough sleep.

Honestly, if I accomplish those goals about 50 percent of the time, I'm doing great. But

I can't fit all these activities in all the time because:

>> I have visitors.

>> I go on trips or vacations.

>> I get overwhelmed with work.

>> A friend or family member needs my immediate help or attention.

>> I get sick or tired.

>> The weather is horrible.

>> The car makes a weird noise, and I have to take it in.

>> Something in the house breaks and I have to wait for a worker.

>> I have an appointment with my accountant, dentist, doctor, or therapist.

We all do the best we can. The key is to ask yourself what your priorities are. Of course, you have to take care of the basic necessities required to get by, pay the bills, put food on the table, keep the house and car running, and so on.

But in addition to those basics, try to fit in one or two of the self-care activities that help you manage anxiety best. For me, it's walking the dog — it's good for me, and I get the reward of a happy dog. For you, it may be something else. The key is to figure out what works for you.

On the days I'm able to stick to a routine, I celebrate the privilege. Don't blame yourself when life interferes — just do what you can do each day.

What Role Does Exercise Play in Reducing Anxiety?

Exercise is the number-one anxiety reducer. It's quick, it takes no planning or equipment, and it works immediately. How many times have you not wanted to work out, but somehow you found a bit of motivation and you felt totally better after?

Working out increases the body's natural *endorphins,* the feel-good chemicals. It reduces anxiety, depression, and pain, and improves overall mood. Any kind of exercise that increases your heart rate and challenges you helps. Find one that you enjoy, and just do it!

TIP

Even bursts of three to five minutes throughout the day can reduce anxiety and improve well-being. Try:

» Doing ten jumping jacks

» Doing a wall sit for two minutes

» Doing ten push-ups

» Taking a five-minute brisk walk

» Going up and down stairs for three minutes

Everyone can incorporate exercise into the day no matter how busy they are. While you're talking on the phone, walk around your house or office. Take a minute at your desk to stand up and sit down five times without using your hands. Keep moving to stay calm!

What Role Does Diet Play in Managing Anxiety?

Anxiety and diet have a complicated relationship. Sometimes a bit of sugar can make you feel better, but that only lasts for a little while. The initial spike in blood sugar eventually leads to a dip in blood sugar, which can ultimately increase anxiety.

A diet full of vegetables, fruits, and whole grains supports steady blood sugar levels. Common-sense good nutrition keeps your body running smoothly.

There's nothing wrong with a cup or two of coffee in the morning, but caffeine can induce anxiety when overdone. Alcohol, which may give you a sense of relaxation in the short term, can interfere with sleep and lead to increased anxiety when you consume too much.

Does Listening to Music Help Anxiety?

Taste in music is highly individual. Some people may relax to the sounds of heavy metal, while others prefer jazz or classical. Whatever works for you is fine. That said, if you're trying to use music to help with anxiety, it should be relaxing, not invigorating. Save the dance music for the dance floor.

TIP

Make an anxiety playlist. Choose songs that soothe you, not ones that make you sad or energized. As long as you're making a playlist, how about one to exercise by? It always helps to find a good beat to keep you moving — and after exercising, you'll also have less anxiety!

How Can I Improve My Sleep to Reduce Anxiety?

Good sleep is essential for mental and physical health. Try to set a regular bedtime and wake-up time. Limit screentime before bed.

I like to read my e-reader before bed. I checked it out to see if using my e-reader was considered "screen time." Apparently, e-readers often use e-ink, which reflects light instead of generating light. So, go ahead and do a bit of reading on your e-reader before bed. But skip the phone or tablet, because they emit blue light, which can interfere with good sleep.

TIP

Here are some other tips for getting a good night's sleep:

» Limit or don't consume caffeine for several hours prior to bed.

» Have no more than one alcoholic drink, preferably with dinner and not later.

» Don't eat a large meal shortly before bed.

» Limit loud noises.

» Keep your room cool if possible.

>> Don't work or eat in your bed. Use your bed only for sleep and sex.

If you wake up for more than ten minutes in the middle of the night, get out of bed and do something boring — don't use a device that emits blue light. Do the dishes or sweep the floor. Go back to bed when you feel sleepy. For more information, see *Sleep For Dummies,* by Clete A. Kushida (Wiley).

What Are the Benefits of Nature for Anxiety?

Numerous studies have shown that being outside in nature reduces stress, improves mood, and leads to better physical health. What an easy way to decrease anxiety!

So, why doesn't everyone do it? Even in cities there are usually a few parks nearby. People with anxiety are often reluctant to get moving, leave their homes, or take the time to just walk or relax outside.

Research shows that spending a couple of hours a week outside may be enough. That may seem overwhelming if you're struggling, so break it down. Aim for 30 minutes a week, broken down into three 10-minute outings. Then slowly increase the amount of time.

Find a buddy to walk with you if possible, or just take a slow walk around the block or down the road. Let the sunshine do its work or the clouds soothe your soul.

Chapter **13**

Social Support and Self-Care

You may be stressed and aggravated by your family or friends from time to time, but considerable research has demonstrated that good close relationships greatly enhance people's sense of well-being. Connections lead to better mental and physical health. Strong connections provide a place to vent and release tension. Close relations can also reduce social isolation and build self-esteem. They also keep your brain in better shape as you get older.

How Can I Establish a Social Support Network to Cope with Anxiety?

Anxiety sometimes makes you want to withdraw and just be by yourself. That's okay once in a while. But social support can provide much-needed relief and distraction. In addition, having others around brings more pleasure into your life.

TIP

Nurture bonds with family, friends, and your community. Have a potluck dinner with your neighbors or your family. Contact a friend you haven't seen for a while and get together for coffee. Take walks in the neighborhood on nice days and chat with people you may not know very well.

TIP

Consider volunteering in your community. Volunteering is a great way to build self-esteem, as well as develop lasting friendships.

Can Setting Boundaries Reduce Anxiety?

Piling too much on your plate makes you anxious, right? Well, if you already have a problem with anxiety, over-scheduling, expecting too much from yourself, and never being able to say no will only make it worse. If you're anxious, it's difficult to stand up for yourself and extremely hard to say "no."

When you have too much pressure, you may add frustration to your anxiety, a bad combination. Spend some time thinking about situations that you find yourself being taken advantage of; then decide to change your behavior. Here are a few ideas for saying no:

» Sorry, that doesn't work for me right now.

» I'd like to help, but it's impossible for me.

» No, thank you, but it sounds like fun.

» It won't work with my schedule.

» I can't do that.

» No.

How Do I Talk to My Family and Friends about My Anxiety?

If you have an anxiety disorder, there is nothing to be ashamed of. Feel free to tell your friends — but also consider who you're talking to. Is it the neighborhood or office gossip? Is it your disapproving aunt?

TIP

Make sure that the people you talk to are trusted friends and family. Then simply be honest. Share with them your symptoms and triggers. If you're getting treatment, talk about the strategies that work best to help you get through your struggles. Sometimes therapists encourage clients to get a coach to help with some exposure exercises (see Chapter 14 for more on exposure therapy).

How Can I Talk to My Children about Anxiety?

First, consider the age of the child. Preschool children and toddlers aren't developmentally prepared to understand the concept of mental health struggles. But by the time kids reach the middle grades of elementary school, most of them have some ideas about feelings.

Talk to your child honestly and sincerely. Tell them what's going on and what triggers your issues. Encourage them to ask questions, and let them know that you're getting help. By being open, you reduce the stigma of mental health problems and give them permission to talk to you when they're confused.

TIP

If your child is anxious, be sure to normalize their feelings and encourage them to discuss any symptoms they may be experiencing. If anxiety is interfering with school, friendships, or relationships, talk to your child's pediatrician and get a referral to a mental health professional.

What Strategies Work Best for Managing Anxiety in Social Situations?

Come up with a plan to increase your social participation. Identify a few situations that you want to start with, such as a neighborhood gathering, a family or work function, a spiritual group, or a hobby group.

Before heading into the situation, take a few deep breaths. Put a soft smile on your face. Remember that others feel the same way you do — you aren't alone.

Find someone who's standing by themselves. Approach and introduce yourself. Ask a general question depending on the setting. Questions can be simple:

» What brings you here today?

» Where are you from?

» What's going on in your life?

TIP

Be a terrific listener. People love to tell stories about themselves. Keep an interested face, nod, breathe, and try to relax. Battle those negative thoughts. You can do this!

What Strategies Can I Use to Communicate My Needs at Work or School due to Anxiety?

Anxiety is a very treatable mental health disorder. The goal of treatment is to reduce symptoms so that they can be tolerated. Therefore, in some ways, accommodations at school or work may be self-defeating. That's because gradual exposure to what makes you anxious is part of most treatments (for more on this subject, turn to Part 4).

Nevertheless, some strategies that may help are part-time work, remote work, work in a quiet setting, noise-cancelling headphones, and flexible scheduling. If anxiety gets in the way of processing information, clear written communication of expectations may be appropriate.

All accommodations, whether at school or work, should be based on your individual needs.

4

Getting Treatment for Anxiety

This part focuses on getting professional help for anxiety. It explains how anxiety is diagnosed and how therapy can help. It introduces different types of therapy and what to expect from your first appointment. Finally, it walks through medications used to treat anxiety and explores other options, including natural remedies, biofeedback, and more.

DID YOU KNOW?

Have you ever seen someone hyperventilating (a symptom of anxiety) and being given a paper bag to blow into? Ever wonder why a paper bag helps? There's nothing magical about a paper bag. The technique works by getting the hyperventilating person to pay attention to their breathing, which usually slows it down.

Chapter **14**
Therapeutic Approaches

Are you thinking about getting help with your problematic anxiety? The first step is getting ready to act. Start to make a plan for change. This chapter details some of the questions you may have about treatment approaches, how to find a good therapist, and what to expect in therapy.

When Should I Seek Professional Help for Anxiety?

There are three questions to consider when deciding to seek professional help:

» **Is your anxiety persistent?** Problematic anxiety isn't one reaction to a stressful event; instead, it lasts longer than expected. For example, a person develops anxiety after a traffic accident, but the anxiety lingers and evolves into a fear of driving.

» **Is your anxiety excessive?** The level of anxiety seems out of proportion to any specific event. For example, someone with anxiety may become extremely anxious when their partner or teenager is a few minutes late getting home.

» **Does your anxiety impair your functioning in some way?** Anxiety may prevent you from attending school or work, taking care of yourself or others, or otherwise perform the normal responsibilities of your daily life. For instance, someone with *agoraphobia* (fear of leaving home) is unable to work because of extreme anxiety.

How Are Anxiety Disorders Diagnosed?

Anxiety disorders are diagnosed by mental health professionals. The provider will ask multiple questions about symptoms of anxiety and triggers for anxiety. They'll also consider persistence, the level of anxiety, and how much the anxiety is impacting day-to-day life.

The diagnosis also involves taking a history of other times you may have had anxiety, whether your family members have anxiety (and, if so, what types), as well as your trauma history.

TIP

It's always important to have a well-trained mental health professional conduct a thorough assessment to obtain an accurate diagnosis.

What Types of Therapy Are Best for Anxiety?

A wide variety of treatment options are available. The following are the most common and based on scientific evidence:

» **Cognitive therapy:** Focuses on teaching new ways of thinking. People with anxiety have distortions in how they perceive events. Usually, they consider events to be more risky or dangerous than they really are.

» **Behavior therapy:** Teaches new ways to approach situations or behave when faced with anxiety. For example, you learn to gradually approach something you fear.

» **Cognitive behavioral therapy (CBT):** Combines cognitive and behavioral approaches and is probably the most common and well-researched approach for treating anxiety.

» **Acceptance and commitment therapy (ACT):** Includes learning to be more mindful and accepting difficult feelings.

There are many other approaches that may be effective at decreasing anxiety, but the ones I list here are strongly supported by multiple research studies.

Exposure is typically part of the treatment of anxiety. *Exposure* involves gradually approaching the feared object or situation. For example, someone who is afraid of dogs would first look at pictures of dogs; then perhaps go to a pet store and look at dogs in kennels; then hold stuffed dogs; then pet a small, calm dog; and gradually walk next to a dog. They would repeat each step until they no longer fear the object. These sessions would take several weeks or months to complete.

Similarly, someone who is afraid to leave their home would start by sitting on the front porch, then walking down the sidewalk, and then walking down the street.

How Do I Find a Therapist?

You may want to start with your primary-care provider. They can refer you to a therapist. If they don't have any names, your insurance company or a trusted friend or family member may give you ideas.

Most professional organizations such as state psychology, state social work, or state counselor associations have websites that list those providers available for therapy. You can also call your local university for potential providers.

After you select a potential provider, contact them. Check to see if their hours will suit you, if they're covered by your insurance, when they can see you, and how soon they're available. Finally, ask them what approach they take to treating anxiety and their experience in this area.

How Can I Prepare for Therapy?

Take some time to think about your symptoms of anxiety. Therapy can move quicker if you've sorted through your symptoms and what seems to trigger them. That way, your therapist can get an idea about what to focus on.

What are the specific goals you have to work on in therapy? For example, do you feel anxious when you have to do something in front of others? Or are you afraid when you're alone? Are you afraid of flying? Driving? Or are do you just generally feel anxious all the time?

What Should I Expect during My First Appointment?

During your first appointment, expect to be asked lots of questions. Your mental health provider will ask you about your current issues, as well as your past mental health problems. In addition, they'll likely ask you to talk briefly about your family, your childhood, your education, and your job experiences.

You should feel comfortable with your therapist. They're trying, in a short time, to get to know you and figure out a treatment plan. Often, the specific plan can take a couple of sessions, especially if you have a difficult problem or an extensive history of mental illness.

Chapter **15**

Medication and Other Treatments

Psychotherapy is the treatment of choice for anxiety. However, medications and other treatments may provide extra help. This chapter takes a look at various treatment options.

Can Medication Help with Anxiety Symptoms?

Yes, medication can reduce anxiety symptoms. Discuss all options with your provider. Medication should be considered when:

» Anxiety severely interferes with functioning.

» Psychotherapy is not available or feasible.

» Psychotherapy has been tried but hasn't been successful.

» Serious depression accompanies anxiety.

» Your physician insists because of health concerns (such as high blood pressure).

» A sudden traumatic event occurs. (Medication may offer immediate relief.)

What Are the Downsides of Anxiety Medications?

Some people feel strongly that they don't want to take medications. They believe that all medications for mental illness are unnecessary. Other downsides include the following:

» **Possible addiction:** Some medications are highly addictive.

» **Long-term effects:** A few medications for anxiety can lead to tremors or weight gain, leading to diabetes.

>> **Side effects:** Introducing new medication to your body can result in side effects. Most of these side effects go away after a few weeks. However, if stomach upset, headaches, dry mouth, dizziness, or sexual dysfunction continue, talk to your healthcare provider.

Talk to your healthcare provider if you have concerns about any of these side effects. Also, if you're breastfeeding, pregnant, or planning to become pregnant, be sure to mention this to your healthcare provider — only a few medications are okay to take when you're pregnant or breastfeeding.

Are There Any New Treatments for Anxiety?

Many *digital therapeutics* (software-based mental health treatments) have been developed to treat anxiety. DaylightRx is the first to be FDA-approved. This digital therapy is prescribed by a healthcare provider. It helps you to learn cognitive behavior therapy (CBT) skills as a way to improve the symptoms related to generalized anxiety disorder. About 70 percent of people using this tool reported a significant reduction in symptoms, even after six months.

Virtual reality (VR) is currently being used to treat anxiety, particularly phobias. VR immerses the person in realistic settings in which they can experience their fears via a headset. Fears can be approached slowly and with deliberate precision using VR.

There are also various brain current stimulations that are used to target severe depression and anxiety that don't respond to the usual treatment. Areas of the brain are targeted by electric or magnetic stimulation. This technique has been primarily used for depression, but has sometimes been found to be successful for anxiety.

New drugs are always being developed. More research is needed, but supervised use of various psychedelics such as lysergic acid diethylamide (LSD) or mushrooms are promising treatments.

Talk to your provider for more information about treatments that you're curious about.

TIP

Are There Natural Remedies for Anxiety?

Natural does not always mean better or more effective. Some supplements and vitamins can interact with prescription medications; others may not be good for you because of health concerns. Talk to your provider to make sure that any natural remedies you're considering are safe for you.

Here are some common supplements and herbal remedies for anxiety:

» B vitamins, especially B6 or B12
» Vitamin D

- Magnesium
- Kava
- L-theanine
- Chamomile
- Lemon balm
- Valerian
- Saint John's wort
- Lavender
- Cannabidiol (CBD), a component of cannabis

Talk to your provider about possible reasons *not* to take these supplements. And keep in mind that alcohol can interact with some supplements or herbs. Report all side-effects to your provider.

How Does Biofeedback Help with Anxiety?

Biofeedback, performed by a trained professional, involves measuring your heart rate, muscle tension, and breathing. The professional then helps you become aware of these involuntary functions and gradually learn to change them.

Biofeedback takes multiple sessions and practice in order to achieve relief from anxiety. With practice, you can use the skills you learn during biofeedback when you're feeling anxious. Biofeedback training is usually provided in addition to psychotherapy.

Can Art, Music, or Pet Therapy Be Effective in Treating Anxiety?

Art, music, and pet therapy can be effective, but they're most often used in concert with psychotherapy or medication. They all can have a calming effect and improve mood. Art and music therapy also involves expression of emotions, which decreases distress. Pet therapy, usually with dogs, can reduce social isolation and loneliness. Interestingly, these therapies are frequently used for hospitalized patients and patients with chronic pain.

How Long Does Treatment for Anxiety Usually Last?

There is no one answer for how long treatment lasts. Many factors go into the decision-making process of the mental health provider, such as:

» How long has the anxiety been present?

» Do you have other mental health problems as well?

» Are you using or abusing substances?

» What sort of stress is part of your life?

For some uncomplicated cases (honestly, the minority), a treatment can last as little as 12 or 16 sessions. But most people take a bit longer because of the complications of everyday life. However, after a dozen sessions you should see significant improvement in your life, even if your treatment isn't finished.

How Can I Stay Motivated during Treatment?

First, remind yourself why you started therapy. Was it to feel less anxious? Or to improve your relationships? Whatever the reason for starting, keep that in mind. Make sure to stay focused on your goal. Of course, your goal may have changed — in that case, remind yourself of your new goal and hang in there.

For most people, therapy becomes a treasured time. Yes, there is work involved and difficult emotions to explore. But when else has one person completely focused on *you?* For an hour each week, you're the star of the show. What a privilege.

What Should I Do If My Treatment Isn't Working?

If you find that treatment isn't really working, make an appointment with your therapist to discuss your concerns. You may be right. Here are a few reasons this may occur:

» You've been unable to establish a therapeutic relationship with your therapist.

In other words, for whatever reason, you just don't click.

» Your therapist reminds you of someone in your past or present life (for example, your father, mother, or kid brother).

» You've been inconsistent about doing homework or coming to sessions.

» You don't feel ready to change.

» You have a terrible therapist (not usually true, but a possibility).

Just because therapy isn't working right now doesn't mean there isn't hope for the future. After you talk to your therapist, you may decide to change therapists or stop treatment for a while (see the next section on how to advocate for yourself).

How Can I Advocate for Myself in the Healthcare System?

The most important task of advocacy is to become educated about the condition that you're seeking care for. Learn about evidence-based treatments for your specific challenge. You can find this information on trusted sites such as:

» **American Academy of Family Physicians:** www.aafp.org

» **American Psychiatric Association:** www.psychiatry.org

- » **American Psychological Association:** www.apa.org
- » **Harvard Health Publishing:** www.health.harvard.edu
- » **Johns Hopkins Medicine:** www.hopkinsmedicine.org
- » **MedlinePlus:** https://medlineplus.gov
- » **National Institutes of Health:** www.nih.gov
- » **U.S. Centers for Disease Control and Prevention:** www.cdc.gov
- » **World Health Organization:** www.who.int

Get in touch with your insurance company and ask for covered providers' names. Mental health treatment is covered by most insurance policies, and you're entitled to get the care you need.

Finally, ask questions. Be assertive. Take notes and ask for clarification when you don't understand something. You deserve to get the treatment you need.

Can Anxiety Be Completely Cured?

Anxiety is an important emotion that alerts our brains and bodies to the possibility that something potentially dangerous is going to happen. That danger signal is a critical response that will never go away.

However, chronic, severe, and life-impacting anxiety can be successfully treated. Those with an anxiety disorder overreact to things that may not be dangerous at all or may just be small glitches in the road. When anxiety is treated, the anxiety response is reserved for occasions that deserve it, such as a lion lurking outside the tent or a hurricane on the horizon. Normal anxiety allows you to take precautions, such as calling animal control or boarding up your windows. You wouldn't want to lose that.

Index

fight-or-flight response, 12, 24

financial stress, 54–55

food, 45, 79

friends, 84–86

G

GAD. *See* generalized anxiety disorder

gender differences in anxiety, 41

generalized anxiety disorder (GAD), 7, 58, 99

genetics, and anxiety, 19

gratitude journal, 71

H

habits, as cause of anxiety, 50–51

Happify (mobile app), 72

Harvard Health Publishing, 105

Headspace (mobile app), 72

heart disease, 29, 47

herbal remedies, 100–101

high blood pressure, 28

hormones, 27–28, 46
  and anxiety, 35, 44
  imbalances, 29

hydration, 46

hyperthyroidism, 29, 47

hypoglycemia, 47

I

IBS. *See* irritable bowel syndrome

impact of anxiety
  on appetite and eating, 14–15
  on attention, 14
  on cognitive functioning, 13
  on concentration, 14
  on decision-making, 13–14
  long-term effects of untreated anxiety, 12
  on memory, 14

insurance, 105

irritability, 58

irritable bowel syndrome (IBS), 26–27

J

Johns Hopkins Medicine, 105

journaling, 71

L

lifestyle, 75
  as cause of anxiety, 50–51
  daily routine, 76–77

risk factors for anxiety,
17–18

  cycle of anxiety, 18

  development of anxiety,
18–19

  genetics, 19

  temperament, 20

  trauma, 20

  upbringing, 19–20, 42

role models, 42

Rootd (mobile app), 72

S

school, communication of
your needs at, 88

screen time, 80

selective mutism, 41

self-advocacy, 104–105

self-care, 77, 87–88

self-confidence, 73

self-esteem, 61, 73,
83, 84

self-help, 69–70

  journaling and expressive
writing, 71

  mobile apps, 72

  self-confidence, 73–74

separation anxiety,
40–41

side effects of anxiety
medications, 99

sleep, 66, 79

  and anxiety, 25, 46

  improving, 80–81

social anxiety disorder, 8, 34,
41, 58

social media, 51–52

social participation, 87

social phobia. *See* social
anxiety disorder

social pressure, 53

social stigma, 41

social support, 83, 84

  talking to children about
anxiety, 86

  talking to friends/family
about anxiety, 85–86

specific phobia, 8

steroids, 62

stimulant medications, 62

stomach problems, 26–27

stress, 34, 50, 53–54

  financial, 54–55

  work-related, 55

subconscious anxiety, 26

substance abuse, 41, 61

sugar, 45, 79

supplements, 100–101

About the Author

Laura L. Smith, PhD, is an author and a clinical psychologist. She is a past president of the New Mexico Psychological Association. Laura has worked in private practice, within hospital settings, and as a consultant for schools. She has presented workshops on cognitive therapy and mental health issues to national and international audiences.

Laura is the author *of Narcissism For Dummies; Anxiety & Depression Workbook For Dummies,* 2nd Edition; *Obsessive Compulsive Disorder For Dummies,* 2nd Edition; and *Anger Management For Dummies,* 3rd Edition (all published by Wiley). She is coauthor with her late husband, Dr. Charles Elliott, of *Quitting Smoking & Vaping For Dummies; Borderline Personality Disorder For Dummies,* 2nd Edition; *Child Psychology & Development For Dummies; Seasonal Affective Disorder For Dummies;* and *Depression For Dummies,* 2nd Edition (all published by Wiley).

Dedication

Coping after significant loss sometimes seems impossible. I had the privilege of a long career teaching others to survive and flourish during their own hardships. My ability to move forward through my own loss was in great part due to the inspiration of others. To my family, the many friends in my village, and the science of psychology, I dedicate this book.

Publisher's Acknowledgments

Senior Managing Editor:
Kristie Pyles

Associate Editor:
Elizabeth Stilwell

Editor: Elizabeth Kuball

Production Editor:
Magesh Elangovan

Cover Design and Image:
Wiley

Special Help:
Carmen Krikorian